ENDOMETRIOSIS SURGERY RECOVERY DIET

Proven Surgical Solutions And Nourishing Your Healing Journey For Reproductive Organ

DR LUCAS KAYCE

DISCLAIMER

This book about illness and nutrition is not meant to replace expert medical advice, diagnosis, or treatment; rather, it is meant purely for informational reasons. This book's content is founded on broad concepts and recommendations for managing diseases and nutrition.

Before adopting any major dietary or lifestyle changes, readers are recommended to speak with a qualified healthcare provider, such as a licensed physician or registered dietitian, especially if they have pre-existing medical concerns. Everybody has different health demands, so what works for one person might not work for another.

The use of the information provided in this book may have unfavorable repercussions or consequences, for which the author and publisher disclaim all liability. No disease is meant to be identified, treated, cured, or prevented by the information provided.

The book may include contain references to medical literature or research findings; however readers are urged to independently confirm this material and contact reliable sources.

It is important to remember that the fields of nutrition and medicine are always changing, and that new findings could have an impact on the advice offered in this book. As a result, readers are urged to keep up with the most recent advancements in healthcare and, when in doubt, seek professional counsel.

By reading this book, readers agree that they are in charge of their own health decisions and release the author and publisher from any liability arising from the use of the material in the book, whether direct or indirect.

TABLE OF CONTENTS

ABOUT THE BOOK

To address a crucial part of women's health, the book "Endometriosis Surgery Recovery Diet" focuses on the role that nutrition plays in the healing process following endometriosis surgery. To fully appreciate the complexity of endometriosis, one must have a thorough understanding of the illness, its causes, and the function of surgery. The book's customized recovery diet is intended to be used in conjunction with surgery to provide a comprehensive healing strategy.

The book walk readers through the period leading up to surgery, stressing the value of speaking with medical specialists and providing preoperative nutrition recommendations.

It goes into great detail about post-surgery diet, emphasizing how important nutrition is to the healing process. This lays the groundwork for the other chapters, which focus on different facets of the recovery diet.

Understanding the influence of hormones and inflammation on endometriosis, the book discusses anti-inflammatory and hormone-balancing diets. Readers are equipped with useful information, recipes, and meal ideas to help them make educated dietary decisions. The relationship between endometriosis and gut health is examined, and suggestions for adding probiotics and prebiotics to the recovery diet are provided.

Furthermore, the book acknowledges the significance of diet in the management of pain and inflammation, explaining pain-relieving foods, herbal medicines, and mindful eating techniques. With chapters devoted to lifestyle and exercise and diet planning and preparation, the book provides a thorough overview for navigating the rehabilitation process.

It emphasizes the value of social and emotional support and offers methods for creating a network of allies and handling difficult emotions. Furthermore, the book foresees and tackles any roadblocks, advising readers to customize the diet to their requirements and see a physician.

"Endometriosis Surgery Recovery Diet" is essentially a helpful tool that provides a methodical and useful approach to nutrition during the healing phase, finally leading to better results and the general health of those who are coping with endometriosis.

CHAPTER ONE

ENDOMETRIOSIS SURGERY RECOVERY DIET OVERVIEW

RECUPERATIVE DIET FOR ENDOMETRIOSIS SURGERY

Endometriosis is a complicated and frequently crippling illness that primarily affects people who are classified as female at birth and affects the reproductive system. Studying endometriosis's definition, causes, and current treatment options is crucial to understanding the condition's subtleties.

This complex illness develops when the endometrium, or tissue resembling the uterine lining, begins to proliferate outside of the uterus.

The symptoms of this abnormal development can be quite severe, greatly affecting the quality of life for those who experience it. These symptoms can include irregular menstruation, pelvic pain, and infertility.

KNOWING WHAT ENDOMETRIOSIS IS

Recognizing the aberrant development of endometrial-like tissue outside of the uterus, such as in the fallopian tubes, ovaries, and pelvic cavity lining, is essential to understanding endometriosis. Hormonal fluctuations cause this ectopic tissue to react, leading to inflammation, scarring, and adhesion formation. The degree of symptoms can differ amongst individuals; some may be in constant agony, while others may show no symptoms at all. Recognizing the variability of endometriosis is essential since individual differences in symptoms and effects might occur.

MEANING AND REASONS

The presence of endometrial tissue outside the uterus is the defining characteristic of endometriosis, although its precise etiology is still unknown. Several ideas, such as retrograde menstruation, which involves the movement of menstrual blood including endometrial cells back into the pelvic cavity, seek to explain the genesis of endometriosis. The development of endometriosis is also influenced by immune system malfunction, genetic predisposition, and environmental factors. To effectively manage and treat this mysterious ailment, a thorough understanding of the interactions between hormones, genetics, and outside variables is frequently necessary.

THE FUNCTION OF SURGERY IN THE TREATMENT OF ENDOMETRIOSIS

In the treatment of endometriosis, surgery is essential, particularly when less intrusive approaches like medication and lifestyle modifications don't work. Laparoscopic excision is a minimally invasive surgical method that is frequently used to remove cysts, adhesions, and endometrial implants. The goals of surgical intervention are to improve overall quality of life, promote fertility, and relieve discomfort. Surgery may not be a one-size-fits-all option, but it is important to remember, that the choice to have surgery should be taken after consulting with medical professionals and taking the patient's unique situation and treatment objectives into account.

THE VALUE OF A CUSTOMIZED REHAB DIET

One cannot stress the need for a specific recovery diet in the management of endometriosis. To support general health and reduce symptoms, nutrition is essential. A few dietary decisions might help reduce symptoms, such as including anti-inflammatory foods, controlling estrogen levels with certain nutrients, and avoiding potential triggers. It is essential to work with healthcare providers, such as nutritionists and dietitians, to customize a recovery diet that takes into account each patient's unique needs and dietary sensitivity to maximize treatment effectiveness and improve the general health of endometriosis patients.

CHAPTER TWO

GETTING READY FOR SURGERY

CONSULTATION WITH MEDICAL SPECIALISTS

Speaking with medical experts is an essential part of getting ready for surgery. This first meeting is crucial because it gives patients a thorough grasp of the process, associated risks, and anticipated results. Patients can talk to their healthcare provider about any worries or inquiries they may have at this stage. Trust is built and expectations are managed when there is open communication between the patient and the medical staff.

Surgeons, anesthesiologists, nurses, and other medical personnel are essential in assisting patients during surgery. They analyze the patient's general health, give important information regarding the procedure, and describe the necessary preparatory measures. Additionally, this visit enables a comprehensive assessment of any prior medical histories or prescription drugs that may affect the surgical operation. This step of the process involves information exchanges that guarantee the patient is informed and psychologically ready for the approaching surgery.

NUTRITIONAL ADVICE PRIOR TO SURGERY

A key component of getting ready for surgery is eating well, and following preoperative dietary recommendations is critical to getting the best results. In the days preceding surgery, medical experts frequently give detailed advice about dietary restrictions. To reduce the risk of problems both during and after the procedure, these instructions may include prohibitions on specific foods and beverages.

Before surgery, patients are usually instructed not to eat solid foods for a predetermined amount of time. Clear liquids up to a specific period before the treatment, like broth and water, may be allowed. These dietary limitations are put in place to lessen the possibility of aspiration while under anesthesia and to facilitate a quicker recovery.

Patients must strictly adhere to these instructions to guarantee that their bodies are suitably ready for the surgical procedure.

PSYCHOLOGICAL AND EMOTIONAL READINESS

There is more to preparing for surgery than just getting physically ready; mental and emotional preparation is just as important. Anxiety, fear, and tension are just a few of the feelings that can surface before surgery. For the patient's general well-being, it is essential to recognize and deal with these feelings. To reduce anxiety and foster a positive outlook, mental readiness is frequently emphasized by healthcare practitioners.

To reduce tension and foster peace, patients are urged to use relaxation methods like deep breathing exercises or meditation. It might also be helpful to discuss any worries or fears honestly and openly with medical specialists. Understanding the surgical procedure, envisioning a positive result, and building resilience are all part of mental preparation.

An important factor in the mental and emotional preparation for surgery is the support that comes from friends and family. During the preoperative phase, having a solid support network can be consoling and reassuring. Overall, a happy experience and a quicker recovery are made possible by mental and emotional preparation, which is a crucial part of the holistic approach to surgery.

CHAPTER THREE

BASICS OF POST-SURGERY NUTRITION

THE ROLE OF NUTRITION IN HEALING

To promote the best possible healing and rehabilitation following surgery, proper nutrition is essential. During surgery, the body is put under a lot of stress, so it's critical to maintain tissue repair, lower inflammation, and improve overall recovery with a well-balanced diet. Sufficient nutrition not only helps the body heal physically but also strengthens the immune system, reducing the risk of infections and other issues after surgery.

AN OVERVIEW OF THE RECOVERY DIET AFTER ENDOMETRIOSIS SURGERY

A specific diet becomes especially significant during the recovery period following endometriosis surgery. A disorder known as endometriosis occurs when tissue that resembles the lining of the uterus grows outside of it. A focused approach to nutrition can help with symptom management, inflammation reduction, and a faster recovery from the physically demanding nature of endometriosis surgery.

The Endometriosis Surgery Recovery Diet emphasizes the use of foods with anti-inflammatory qualities to reduce pain and discomfort related to the condition. Flaxseeds, walnuts, and fatty fish are among the foods high in omega-3 fatty acids that may help lower inflammation. Furthermore, antioxidants—which are present in fruits and vegetables—are essential for promoting the body's natural healing processes.

HARMONIZING ELEMENTS FOR REMEDY

A crucial component of a post-surgery diet is nutritional balancing, which guarantees that the body gets the components it needs for a speedy recovery. Lean protein sources such as fish, chicken, beans, and tofu can help with muscle rebuilding and overall recovery. Proteins are essential for tissue repair and regeneration.

The body needs carbohydrates to perform at its best, and eating a diet high in whole grains, fruits, and vegetables helps sustain energy levels during the recuperation stage.

Although it's sometimes overlooked, staying properly hydrated is just as important for healing. Maintaining hydration is beneficial for several body processes, such as toxin removal, nutrition transfer, and blood circulation. Drinking more water should be monitored and enhanced, particularly if the procedure results in fluid loss or if taking certain medications makes you dehydrated.

Minerals and vitamins are examples of micronutrients that are essential to the healing process. The synthesis of collagen, which is essential for wound healing, is one of vitamin C's well-known functions. Bell peppers, strawberries, and citrus fruits are all great providers of vitamin C. Zinc is another important mineral that helps with tissue regeneration and immunological function. It can be found in meat, dairy, and legumes.

The idea of post-surgery nutrition is complex and has multiple facets. Its significance is highlighted by its ability to promote healing, control symptoms, and avert problems. Dietary modifications for particular surgical procedures—like endometriosis surgery—can improve the effectiveness of the healing process. Balancing nutrients, staying hydrated, and including foods with anti-inflammatory and healing characteristics are key components of a comprehensive post-surgery diet plan.

CHAPTER FOUR

ANTI-INFLAMMATORY FOODS

UNDERSTANDING INFLAMMATION IN ENDOMETRIOSIS

In the context of endometriosis, inflammation plays a critical role in the evolution and intensity of symptoms associated with this disorder. Endometriosis is a persistent illness where tissue comparable to the lining of the uterus grows outside the uterus. This aberrant tissue growth can lead to inflammation, producing pain, discomfort, and serious consequences. Inflammation in endometriosis is mostly triggered by the immune system's response to the presence of endometrial-like tissue in locations where it shouldn't be. The inflammatory process contributes to the production of adhesions, scar tissue, and the continuous pain experienced by persons with endometriosis.

Understanding the inflammatory nature of endometriosis is key to managing the condition properly.

Anti-inflammatory therapies constitute a major component of the overall therapy regimen. While medicinal interventions are often necessary, food choices can also play a key role in controlling inflammation and reducing symptoms. Incorporating anti-inflammatory items into the diet is a proactive approach that can complement medical therapies and boost overall well-being.

INCORPORATING ANTI-INFLAMMATORY FOODS INTO YOUR DIET

Adopting a diet high in anti-inflammatory foods can be a significant component in treating inflammation linked with endometriosis. Anti-inflammatory foods are those that assist reduce inflammation in the body and may include a variety of fruits, vegetables, whole grains, and specific fats. Fruits and vegetables, particularly those rich in antioxidants and phytochemicals, can help neutralize free radicals and control the inflammatory response.

Berries, leafy greens, and cruciferous vegetables are examples of such anti-inflammatory foods.

Omega-3 fatty acids, present in fatty fish like salmon, walnuts, and flaxseeds, have been shown to have anti-inflammatory benefits. These good fats can help balance the ratio of pro-inflammatory to anti-inflammatory molecules in the body, potentially decreasing the influence of inflammation on endometriosis symptoms. Additionally, herbs and spices such as turmeric and ginger contain chemicals with anti-inflammatory effects and can be added to meals to enhance flavor while delivering potential therapeutic advantages.

Maintaining a well-balanced diet that includes a variety of nutrient-dense foods is vital for general health and may contribute to reducing inflammation.

It's crucial to limit or avoid processed foods, excessive intake of refined carbohydrates, and certain fats that may induce inflammation. Working with a healthcare practitioner or a certified dietitian can assist in customizing dietary suggestions to individual needs and tastes, ensuring a sustainable and successful anti-inflammatory approach.

RECIPES AND MEAL IDEAS

Creating meals that feature anti-inflammatory foods can be both delicious and supportive of controlling endometriosis symptoms. Consider starting the day with a smoothie including antioxidant-rich berries, spinach, and a spoonful of flaxseeds for extra omega-3s. For lunch, a vibrant salad with mixed greens, cherry tomatoes, avocado, and grilled salmon gives a nutrient-packed, anti-inflammatory alternative. Incorporating turmeric and ginger into soups, stews, or stir-fries provides both taste and potential anti-inflammatory benefits.

Quinoa, a whole grain high in protein and fiber, can serve as a base for numerous meals, such as a Mediterranean-inspired bowl with olives, cucumbers, cherry tomatoes, and a drizzle of olive oil. Snacking on walnuts or almonds and sipping herbal teas with anti-inflammatory characteristics throughout the day are other ways to fill the diet with helpful nutrients.

Experimenting with dishes and modifying them to specific taste preferences can make the anti-inflammatory approach to eating pleasurable and sustainable. While nutrition alone may not replace medical therapies, it can add to an overall approach for reducing inflammation and increasing the quality of life for patients with endometriosis.

CHAPTER FIVE

HORMONE-BALANCING FOODS

IMPACT OF HORMONES ON ENDOMETRIOSIS

The role of hormones in endometriosis is a vital component of understanding the disorder. Endometriosis is a medical disorder when tissue comparable to the lining inside the uterus, called endometrium, begins to grow outside the uterus. Hormones, particularly estrogen, have a crucial role in the development and progression of endometriosis. Estrogen is believed to increase the formation of endometrial tissue, and changes in estrogen levels can exacerbate the symptoms of endometriosis, such as pelvic discomfort, heavy menstrual bleeding, and infertility.

Therefore, controlling hormone levels becomes vital in addressing and easing the consequences of endometriosis.

FOODS THAT SUPPORT HORMONE BALANCE

Foods have a vital role in supporting hormone balance, and implementing a hormone-balancing diet can be useful for persons coping with endometriosis. Cruciferous vegetables like broccoli, cauliflower, and Brussels sprouts have chemicals that benefit the liver in metabolizing estrogen, helping to maintain a healthy hormonal balance. Additionally, meals rich in omega-3 fatty acids, such as fatty fish like salmon and flaxseeds, can help reduce inflammation and promote hormone control. Consuming fiber-rich foods, particularly whole grains, legumes, and fruits, aids in estrogen elimination, reducing its reabsorption into the circulation.

SAMPLE HORMONE-BALANCING MEAL PLANS

In developing a hormone-balancing meal plan, it's crucial to focus on nutrient-dense, complete foods that encourage hormonal wellness. A sample meal plan would include a breakfast of overnight oats with flaxseeds and berries, offering a combination of fiber, omega-3 fatty acids, and antioxidants. For lunch, a quinoa salad with a range of colorful vegetables and a piece of grilled salmon can deliver a balanced combination of nutrients supporting hormonal balance. Dinner might consist of roasted Brussels sprouts, broccoli, and a lean protein source like chicken or tofu, giving important ingredients for estrogen metabolism.

In addition to specific foods, paying attention to meal timing and portion control is vital for hormone balance. Eating regular, balanced meals throughout the day helps regulate blood sugar levels, minimizing insulin spikes that can disrupt hormone function.

Avoiding excessive consumption of processed meals, sugary snacks, and refined carbohydrates is also suggested since these might lead to hormone abnormalities.

While dietary treatments are useful, it's crucial to realize that individual responses to food can vary. Consulting with a healthcare expert or a certified dietitian is recommended to adapt a hormone-balancing meal plan to individual needs and guarantee comprehensive management of endometriosis symptoms. Integrating these dietary strategies with other lifestyle modifications and medical interventions can contribute to a holistic approach to managing hormonal imbalances associated with endometriosis.

CHAPTER SIX

GUT HEALTH AND ENDOMETRIOSIS

ENDOMETRIOSIS AND THE GUT RELATIONSHIP

The intricate relationship between gut health and endometriosis has been an area of growing interest in recent years. Endometriosis, a chronic condition characterized by the presence of endometrial-like tissue outside the uterus, can significantly impact a woman's reproductive health. Emerging research suggests a potential link between the gut microbiome and the development or exacerbation of endometriosis. The gut microbiome, consisting of trillions of microorganisms, plays a crucial role in maintaining overall health, regulating immune responses, and influencing hormonal balance.

Studies have revealed alterations in the composition of the gut microbiota in women with endometriosis compared to those without the condition. Imbalances in the gut microbiome may contribute to systemic inflammation, which is a key factor in the pathogenesis of endometriosis. Furthermore, the stomach may act as a reservoir for inflammation, which could cause inflammatory molecules to spread and aggravate endometriotic lesions. Comprehending the complex relationship between the gut and endometriosis provides opportunities to investigate innovative treatment approaches and lifestyle adjustments for better endometriosis management.

GUT HEALTH BENEFITS OF PREBIOTICS AND PROBIOTICS

Probiotics, also known as "good" or "beneficial" bacteria, are live microorganisms that, when taken in sufficient quantities, have positive effects on health. Through the promotion of a diverse and well-balanced microbial community, these microorganisms can have a positive impact on the gut microbiome. Adding probiotics to one's diet may help regulate the inflammatory response and support immune system balance in the context of endometriosis.

It has been demonstrated that some probiotic strains have anti-inflammatory qualities, which may help to lessen the systemic inflammation brought on by endometriosis.

Conversely, prebiotics are indigestible fibers that provide energy to good bacteria in the digestive system. A healthier gut environment can be promoted by including prebiotics in the diet, which can support the growth and activity of probiotics. Prebiotics are abundant in whole foods like fruits, vegetables, and whole grains. Through the combination of probiotics and prebiotics, endometriosis sufferers may increase the variety and quantity of good bacteria in their digestive tract, which may have an impact on the inflammatory environment linked to the disease.

GUT-SOOTHING RECIPES

One holistic strategy that people with endometriosis can think about using to manage their symptoms is to adopt a gut-friendly diet. Including foods that are high in nutrients and reduce inflammation has a positive effect on gut health and general well-being. You can customize a wide range of gut-friendly recipes to meet specific dietary needs and preferences. For instance, meals high in fiber from whole grains, fruits, and vegetables supply vital prebiotics that help a healthy gut flora.

Furthermore, probiotics found in fermented foods like kefir, yogurt, sauerkraut, and kimchi support a varied microbial community. To improve gut health, include these foods as snacks or in your regular meals. Because they may help reduce endometriosis-related inflammation, anti-inflammatory herbs and spices like ginger and turmeric can be added to recipes. In general, following a gut-friendly diet entails choosing foods carefully that support a healthy gut microbiome and nourish the body, which may help manage endometriosis symptoms.

CHAPTER SEVEN

USING DIET TO CONTROL PAIN AND INFLAMMATION

FOODS TO REDUCE PAIN

Eating a diet high in anti-inflammatory foods is an important part of managing pain and inflammation. Including these foods can be crucial for easing discomfort and enhancing general health. Berries, cherries, and leafy greens are examples of fruits and vegetables that are high in antioxidants and can help reduce inflammation. Flaxseeds, walnuts, and fatty fish like salmon are rich sources of omega-3 fatty acids, which are known to have anti-inflammatory qualities that help reduce pain.

Nuts, legumes, and whole grains all contain fiber and vital nutrients that help the body's defense mechanisms against inflammation. Curcumin-containing spice turmeric has strong anti-inflammatory properties and is widely used in cooking. Known for its analgesic and anti-inflammatory qualities, ginger can be added to food or drunk as a tea. Furthermore, green tea's polyphenol content has anti-inflammatory properties, which makes it a useful beverage for people who are managing their pain with diet.

SUPPLEMENTS AND HERBAL REMEDIES:

The ability of herbs and supplements to reduce pain and inflammation has long been known. One of the well-known herbal remedies is Boswellia serrata, which is made from the resin of the Boswellia tree and is frequently used in traditional medicine due to its anti-inflammatory qualities.

Devil's Claw is a different herb that comes from South Africa and has been researched for its anti-inflammatory properties, especially for arthritis.

Omega-3 fatty acid-rich supplements like fish oil have drawn interest for their capacity to control inflammatory reactions. Supplements containing concentrated curcumin extracts, such as turmeric, provide a convenient way to add this potent anti-inflammatory agent to one's daily regimen.

Commonly used for joint health, glucosamine, and chondroitin are thought to help with pain management for conditions like osteoarthritis.

USING MINDFUL EATING TO MANAGE PAIN

The practice of mindful eating, which emphasizes awareness and consciousness while consuming food, can be very helpful in the management of pain. People may become more conscious of how their bodies react to various foods if they focus on the sensory aspects of eating. This strategy entails appreciating every bite, identifying signals of hunger and fullness, and being aware of how particular foods affect general well-being.

Making conscious food choices and focusing on nutrient-dense, anti-inflammatory foods are other aspects of mindful eating. This entails choosing complete, unprocessed foods and preparing meals that feature a range of hues and textures.

By encouraging a nutritious and well-balanced diet, mindful eating techniques may improve the quality of one's relationship with food and lead to better pain management results. This method also helps people become more attuned to their bodies, acknowledging and honoring signals about inflammation and pain.

CHAPTER EIGHT

PLANNING AND PREPARING MEALS

HOW TO MAKE A WEEKLY MENU

Planning your meals is crucial to eating a balanced, healthful diet. It entails carefully planning and arranging a week's worth of meals, taking convenience, taste preferences, and nutritional needs into account. A weekly meal plan has several advantages, including assisting people in choosing better foods, preventing impulsive purchases, and saving time and money. Begin by listing all of the meals for the upcoming week, including breakfast, lunch, dinner, and snacks. Think about including a range of food groups, including whole grains, fruits, vegetables, lean meats, dairy products, and dairy substitutes.

When making a weekly meal plan, consider your obligations and timetable. On days when your schedule is lighter, set aside more time for cooking; on days when it's busy, plan simpler, faster meals.

It's also critical to be adaptable and willing to make changes in response to unanticipated events or shifting tastes. To maintain a varied and engaging menu, try out several foods and cuisines. To save time and reduce food waste, create a shopping list based on the meals you have planned.

<h2 style="text-align:center">RECIPES TO HELP YOU HEAL</h2>

Cooking may be a fulfilling and therapeutic hobby, particularly for people going through recovery. Some cooking techniques can help speed up the healing process, whether you're recuperating from an illness, or surgery, or are just concentrating on your general well-being. Give top priority to foods high in nutrients, such as whole grains, lean meats, and fresh produce, as these will aid in the body's processes of repair and regeneration. To help reduce inflammation, think about adding anti-inflammatory items to your dishes, such as ginger and turmeric.

Make cooking easier by choosing basic, easily digestible foods when recovering from surgery. Make use of culinary methods like roasting, steaming, or slow cooking that take less time and effort to complete. Batch cooking is another great option; create larger quantities of dishes and freeze portions for later use. Include items high in water content in your diet, such as stews, soups, and juicy fruits. Additionally, pay attention to your body's signals and modify meal timing and portion sizes as necessary to maintain a steady level of energy during the healing process.

SIMPLE, HIGH-NUTRIENT RECIPES

In their culinary pursuits, many people aim to create meals that are high in nutrients and simple to make. A broad range of vitamins and minerals is ensured by including a variety of colorful fruits and vegetables in dishes. For instance, a straightforward stir-fry with a variety of veggies and lean protein may be a filling, fast supper. Try using whole grains as the foundation for salads or bowls, such as quinoa, brown rice, or farro, to increase your intake of complex carbohydrates and fiber.

Try experimenting with plant-based proteins like tofu, lentils, and beans for a flexible and simple-to-prepare source of protein. Meals that only require one pot, such as casseroles or chili, make cooking easier and cleaning simpler. Never be afraid to add herbs and spices to improve flavor without adding too much sugar or salt. Smoothies including mixed fruits, greens, and a source of protein are great choices for a quick and nutrient-dense breakfast or snack. These quick dishes, which emphasize nutrition and ease of preparation, add variety and satisfaction to any meal plan.

CHAPTER NINE

EXERCISE AND LIFESTYLE

MODERATE EXERCISES FOR RECOVERY

Whether recovering from an illness, accident, or strenuous physical activity, moderate exercise is essential. These low-impact workouts are made to encourage flexibility, mobility, and general well-being while putting the least amount of strain on the body. Gentle exercise routines include yoga, swimming, and strolling.

Walking helps to improve cardiovascular health without putting undue strain on the joints because of its regular and natural movements. Swimming is a great non-weight-bearing exercise choice for people who want to heal without overstretching their muscles and joints. Furthermore, by emphasizing thoughtful poses and controlled movements, yoga helps promote physical and mental healing while also increasing flexibility and lowering stress.

TECHNIQUES FOR STRESS MANAGEMENT

Stress management has become crucial to preserving general well-being in the fast-paced and demanding world of modern living. There are numerous strategies available to assist people in managing their stress levels. The capacity of mindfulness and meditation techniques to promote focus and calmness has made them more popular.

By encouraging people to live in the present, these methods raise awareness and lessen the negative effects of stress.

Deep diaphragmatic breathing is one of the easy-to-use yet effective breathing exercises that help to calm the nervous system and promote relaxation. Furthermore, hobbies, exercise, and time spent in nature may all serve as powerful stress relievers and provide people a chance to relax and rejuvenate.

INCLUDING HEALTHFUL PRACTICES IN EVERYDAY LIFE

Maintaining long-term health requires incorporating healthy behaviors into daily living. Sustainability is ensured by smoothly integrating healthy behaviors into everyday activities as opposed to treating health as a stand-alone concept. Because both physical and mental health depend heavily on getting enough sleep, it is essential to establish a regular sleep pattern. Eating a diet high in fruits, vegetables, whole grains, and other nutrients and well-balanced foods promotes general vitality.

Frequent exercise, especially in the form of quick workouts spread out throughout the day, improves mood and helps sustain fitness levels. Although it's sometimes overlooked, being hydrated is essential to overall health as it supports several body processes.

Incorporating moments of relaxation, such as quick breaks or mindfulness exercises, can also lessen the negative effects of everyday stressors and promote a well-rounded approach to wellbeing. To create a durable basis for a healthy existence, it is important to cultivate habits that are feasible within one's lifestyle and in line with personal beliefs.

CHAPTER TEN

EMOTIONAL AND SOCIAL ASSISTANCE

CREATING A SUPPORT NETWORK

For those who want to be socially and emotionally well, the idea of creating a support network is essential. A network of people who are there to provide assistance, understanding, and support when things are tough. It's a broad group that could include of coworkers, friends, family, and even local support networks. Creating and sustaining such a network is essential to resilience and a sense of belonging. These relationships act as a safety net for those going through difficult times emotionally by giving them a place to talk about their experiences, get guidance, and be supported.

COPING MECHANISMS FOR EMOTIONAL HEALTH

Coping mechanisms are essential for fostering emotional health. These techniques cover a variety of actions and methods that people can use to successfully manage stress, anxiety, and other emotional difficulties. Emotional resilience can be enhanced by practices like mindfulness, deep breathing exercises, and partaking in enjoyable hobbies or pastimes. Another crucial coping mechanism is to seek out professional assistance, such as counseling or therapy. Building healthy routines, leading a balanced lifestyle, and engaging in self-compassion exercises are essential elements of cultivating emotional well-being.

MAKING CONNECTIONS WITH OTHERS IN THE ENDOMETRIOSIS COMMUNITY

One special and important component of social and emotional support is making connections with others in the Endometriosis community. People who have endometriosis, a chronic medical disorder that affects the reproductive system, may find it emotionally taxing. Making relationships with people who have gone through comparable things helps foster empathy and a sense of community. Endometriosis sufferers have access to online communities, support groups, and social gatherings as means of networking, exchanging ideas, and providing assistance to one another. These relationships dispel the emotions of loneliness that frequently accompany chronic health issues by fostering a sense of empowerment and solidarity.

Creating a support system, embracing coping mechanisms for mental health, and interacting with members of niche communities such as endometriosis are essential elements of an all-encompassing strategy for social and emotional support. These ideas stress the value of connections, self-care, and life experiences in fostering resilience and mental health.

CHAPTER ELEVEN

HANDLING DIFFICULTIES

HANDLING SETBACKS

We all face obstacles and disappointments in life that might throw off our goals and ambitions. Our resilience and capacity to recover are frequently determined by how we handle and recover from these setbacks. Having a growth mentality is essential when dealing with setbacks; instead of seeing them as insurmountable obstacles, you should see them as chances for personal development.

Accepting setbacks as a necessary part of the path enables people to grow more resilient and adaptive.

Recognizing and managing the emotions connected to the task is a useful method for handling setbacks. Letting go of disappointment, irritation, or even a feeling of failure and allowing oneself to feel and comprehend these feelings is an essential first step in recovery. Emotional repression must be avoided as it can impede the healing process.

In addition, failures offer a chance for introspection. Analyzing the elements that led to the failure enables people to pinpoint areas in need of development and make the required adjustments. This process of reflection allows people to grow personally and gives them the knowledge they need to deal with obstacles in the future more skillfully.

CHANGING THE DIET TO MEET INDIVIDUAL NEEDS

While keeping a good, balanced diet is essential for overall well-being, it's also critical to understand that there isn't a single, universally applicable nutritional strategy. Every person has different nutritional needs depending on their age, activity level, metabolism, and medical problems. Therefore, for long-term sustainability and health, dietary adaptation to fit individual demands is crucial.

Understanding and appreciating the variety of dietary options is a fundamental component of customizing a diet to meet the needs of each individual. Foods have varying effects on different bodies, so what suits one individual may not suit another.

It's critical to monitor how each person responds to different foods and modify them as necessary. Being adaptable is essential because it enables adjustments in response to shifting conditions and changing health objectives.

Consulting with a certified dietitian or other nutrition specialist can also offer insightful information about personal dietary needs. These professionals are capable of evaluating dietary preferences, lifestyle, and medical problems to develop customized nutrition regimens. People can make well-informed dietary selections that suit their requirements and objectives by working with professionals.

LOOKING FOR EXPERT ADVICE

Overcoming obstacles frequently calls for a blend of independent work and outside assistance. Getting expert advice is a proactive and successful way to get past challenges in many facets of life. When it comes to mental health concerns, job decisions, or obstacles to personal growth, experts in their domains can offer invaluable perspectives, tactics, and assistance.

In terms of mental health, seeing certified specialists for therapy or counseling can provide a secure setting for exploring feelings, creating coping strategies, and learning more about oneself. To promote mental and emotional well-being, professionals can offer evidence-based interventions and therapy approaches catered to the unique needs of each individual.

Mentoring and professional counseling can be helpful in areas like career growth. The knowledge and counsel of mentors or career counselors can be helpful to professionals looking for career assistance. They can provide insightful viewpoints, networking opportunities, and tactical advice to help traverse the intricacies of the professional landscape.

Getting professional advice is a proactive move toward both personal and professional development since it gives people access to knowledge, opens their eyes to fresh viewpoints, and helps them create effective problem-solving techniques.